THE BEAUTY OF SEX
Unveiling the routes of Pleasure

Valerie C. Hill

Table of contents

<u>**What is sexual exploration?**</u>
<u>**What are the advantages of sexual exploration?**</u>

<u>**What is the difference between sexual exploration and sexual experimentation?**</u>

<u>**Masturbation**</u>

<u>**Shared sexual experiences**</u>

<u>**Sexual fantasy**</u>

<u>**Inspiration for your sexual adventure**</u>

<u>**CHAPTER 5**</u>

<u>**PRIORITIZE SEX**</u>

Introduction

Unveiling the routes of Pleasure" is an appealing investigation of the numerous routes to sensory and interpersonal pleasure. This book takes readers on a thrilling journey, exploring the complexities and complexity of pleasure, connection, and personal growth within the realm of human sexuality.

Through beautiful language and fascinating insights, "Sexual Symphony" celebrates the enormous beauty and complexity of human sexual encounters. It extends beyond the fundamental physical, extending into the emotional, psychological, and spiritual components that connect with our needs.

Each chapter in "sensory Symphony" unveils a new layer of sensory pleasure, from the discovery of self-awareness and self-acceptance to the art of communication and the power of exploration. It gives practical instruction, intelligent exercises, and expert advice to help readers follow their own individual roads to pleasure.

This book acknowledges the plurality of human goals, realizing that fulfillment comes in all forms and expressions. It promotes a sex-positive and inclusive perspective, embracing diverse orientations, identities, and relationship dynamics while urging readers to embrace their genuine selves.

Drawing on a variety of research, personal anecdotes, and insight from renowned experts, "sensual Symphony" examines the changing potential of sensual encounters. It invites readers to form a stronger connection with their bodies, develop greater self-confidence, and cultivate meaningful connections with their partners.

Above all, "Sensual Symphony" reminds readers that fulfillment is a lifelong adventure, a perpetual symphony of sensations, emotions, and connections. It inspires individuals to listen to the melodies within themselves, to embrace the rhythms of desire, and to construct their own unique paths to physical pleasure.

Through its beautiful narrative and deep observations, "Sensual Symphony" delivers a captivating alternative to standard ideas on pleasure and contentment. It invites readers to release the complete spectrum of pleasure and connection, leading to a more vivid, authentic, and rewarding sexual existence.

It is crucial to foster consent, respect, and open communication in all personal encounters.

Building the foundation for your sex apprehensive to put herself in a position of vulnerability by giving herself to him sexually. For her, having sex while feeling emotionally detached may be comparable to having sex with a stranger.

For women, the want to be intimate is more of an "emotional drive," whereas for males, it's more of a bodily need. Husbands typically fail to comprehend the concept that women have to feel emotionally close and comfortable before they can "decide" to have sex. This is especially true given that partners are not made to have to feel emotionally close before they wish to have sex. They also don't have to deliberately "decide" to get there sexually. Their brains and bodies effectively do it for them.

Men typically have enough sexual desire floating about to easily say yes to sex, whether their spouse has been lovely or attentive to them that day or not. For a woman, it isn't that easy to disregard it if her partner has been a jerk that day. It isn't simple to say yes if, in general, her partner merely refuses to acknowledge, respect, and meet her emotional needs in the marriage.

So, men, if you want to "get fortunate," you may want to listen to how connected your wife feels to you and consistently focus on those things that make it easier for her to say yes to sex.

CHAPTER 1

FOUNDATION OF SEX

Building a Foundation for Your Sexuality in Your Relationship

Let's face it, until you have a rock-solid foundation in your relationship with your significant other, you will eventually be on unstable ground. For some, this isn't really a revelation, but for others, it's about truly appreciating what a foundation actually is.

To me, foundation signifies the building blocks of a satisfying relationship and result. And much like a home with frail or seriously broken flooring, roofing, or walls, it can't stand upright or provide protection if the foundation isn't there in the first place.

So when it comes to relationships, it's necessary to develop a framework of understanding, trust, respect, compassion, empathy, vision, cooperation, grace, and forgiveness. Of course, this is something that is established over time, particularly as partnerships may be defined differently as they traverse their paths.

But the foundation has to be the thing that keeps the connection together and withstands the ups and downs. It ultimately boils down to having a common conviction in self-development and spiritual growth, plus acknowledging that you are both on the journey to understanding why you are here on Earth.

Tips regarding how to start constructing or strengthening that foundation

1. Grow Together in Self-Development

If you are both enthusiastic about educating themselves, particularly in areas of self-development and spiritual growth, so that you link more deeply rather than dread intimacy, then that is the basis that you can always come back to. Basically, it's what provides you with the greatest potential for the marriage to have longevity. In addition, multiple studies have indicated that the partnerships and marriages that endure the longest are those where the couples share the same underlying values and views.

2. Create a never-ending honeymoon phase.

Even when the so-called honeymoon phase looks to be ending, there's no reason why it can't continue. But the only way it's going to accomplish this is if:

You have the appropriate views about partnerships.
You realize why you are genuinely getting into the relationship.
Your spouse shares the same basic values as you do.
By its very nature, whether it's monetary stuff, sex, or anything else, everything has a propensity for changing and vanishing in life. So you want to look at methods of returning to the foundation because it's the thing that is immutable and rock-solid.

3. Perceive relationships the right way.

There's no disputing that the worldwide divorce rate is huge. However, I believe that's because there is a false image or ideal about partnerships being like the Cinderella narrative. People have a propensity to project their own needs onto their spouse and assume they are going to fill that hole for them. But it's crucial to know that your spouse is not the one who is going to make you happy; you have to experience that first and foremost. At the end of the day, you're on your own trip, and having a soul buddy share that with you is really a great thing. It's also the proper way to think about having a good, rewarding relationship.

4. Love unconditionally.

A rock-solid relationship is about having no expectations, not judging, and learning about what love actually is, which is unconditional. That is, loving someone but letting them go at the same time. Too frequently, we want to control our spouse, so unconditional love is continuously about loving and letting go, loving and letting go, loving and letting go. It also involves embracing and loving the elements in them that we don't really like.

5. Look within

A lot of the time, your spouse may reflect things back to you that need to be repaired inside yourself. But if you're not willing to look at those things, then you tend to run away. The temptation is to ignore them because you don't want to look at those things in yourself that need to be repaired. In fact, you're more likely to point the blame at your spouse, saying, "It's your issue to sort out." The idea is to look at yourself and observe what's being reflected back, because this is most likely something you need to take responsibility for. Once you perceive it this way, you may look at it as a connection between development and evolution that serves to cement and bring things together.

6. Choose love, not fear.

If we actually come down to it, most of us are terrified of love, even though it's the most beautiful thing around. What's more, there's only true fear or love out there. Having a fear of intimacy comes back to oneself. But it's crucial not to blame this worry on your spouse, including whatever self-worth concerns you may have hidden deep within. As I've mentioned previously, you really need to love yourself first and find out how to fully accept it. Of course, this may be challenging since any fear-based sentiments exist at a deeper level. By recognizing and coming to terms with these feelings, it helps fortify the basis of our connection with ourselves and with others.

Important things to watch out for in a relationship

Every connection is unique. So, although some couples may rank sex at the top of their priority list, others may consider other parts of the relationship more vital.
Partners may not prioritize sex for a variety of reasons.

For example, having a decreased sex desire, being asexual, refraining from sex owing to religious or cultural beliefs, or living with certain physical problems may all play a role.

"Sex is not the only component of the relationship that makes couples happy; it isn't always an essential ingredient for a healthy relationship."

In fact, scientists think the following parts of a relationship may have just as much value as sex, if not more.

1. Emotional security

Emotional stability is the cornerstone of every loving and supportive relationship, according to Jennine Estes, a certified marital and family therapist and founder of Estes Therapy.

Emotional security implies that you feel comfortable enough to be honest and vulnerable in your relationship.

For example, if you feel ignored by your spouse or something they say hurts you, you should feel comfortable discussing why you're unhappy with them without fearing their reply.

In contrast, partners who don't feel emotionally comfortable could become defensive or belligerent during arguments and withdraw, shut down, or avoid fights totally. These actions may inhibit communication and, in some circumstances, generate secret resentments.
To establish emotional security, you might:

Let them know when something they do annoys you, but approach them in a non-accusatory manner so they know you're giving them the benefit of the doubt.
Summarize or reflect back on what they've said to demonstrate you've listened and cared about their views and emotions.
Validate and express empathy for their feelings by stating things such as, "It makes

sense you'd feel sad in that scenario" or "That must've been so difficult. I'd feel the same way."

2. Quality time

A small 2021 study indicated that spending quality time with your spouse, whether simply chatting or engaging in an activity, might improve you:

Feel more fulfilled in the relationship.
Perceive more positive aspects in your connection.
Experience closer intimacy with your companion.
There's no hard-and-fast rule on how much time you should spend together. Ultimately, experts say it's about discovering what works for you, which may mean allocating a stretch of bonding time on weekends, setting aside an hour each day, or conducting date night once a week.

Shared experiences are significant since they may uncover common ground. They may also make you feel like a team, generate pleasant memories to look back on, and inspire you to continue working on the connection.

"The more the couple can break away from everyday stress and be there for one another, the more they will feel connected," Estes adds.

3. Positive interactions

According to a comprehensive study by psychologist John Gottman, couples who had five or more pleasant encounters for each negative one were more likely to remain married than divorce. Using this magic ratio, Gottman could determine whether a couple would remain married with almost 90% accuracy.

Negative interactions may include being too critical or dismissive of your partner's sentiments, raising your voice, or giving them the quiet treatment. These habits may take a toll on the trust, respect, and intimacy in your relationship.

Conversely, you may have more pleasant relationships by:

Showing real interest in your partner's remarks through establishing eye contact, asking open-ended questions, and exercising introspective listening.
Expressing physical love by hugging them when they return home from work, caressing their back while you watch a movie, or holding their hand while on a neighborhood walk

Complimenting them and expressing thanks and appreciation for the things they do to make your life simpler.
Finding things to agree on during a dispute rather than merely concentrating on your differences.

Offering a heartfelt apology after you've done something harmful
Finding methods to laugh together to reduce the tension and lighten the atmosphere during arguments and small conflicts

4. Intimacy

Intimacy cultivates a feeling of proximity. While a lot of people believe intimacy merely implies sex, physical closeness is just one component.

Other equally significant sorts of closeness include:

Mental or intellectual intimacy: This entails learning new things together. For instance, you may recommend joining up for a cooking class or discussing things you both find intriguing.
Emotional intimacy: This entails communicating about your deepest ideas, wishes, and anxieties. You may urge your spouse to do the same by asking open-ended

questions like, "What makes you feel the most loved?" "What is anything you want to do but feel too terrified to undertake?" or "When you're feeling worried, what's the greatest thing I can do for you?"

Experiential intimacy: This might involve any form of partnership. To create this form of connection, you may pick a pastime to discuss or do home repair chores together.

5. Respect

Mutual respect in a relationship may add to feelings of trust and emotional stability and foster more honesty and vulnerability. It may even increase relationship happiness and quality.

You may demonstrate your respect in daily situations by:

- Honoring boundaries
- Giving each other space as required.
- Supporting each other's objectives and interests

- Acknowledging each other as people with distinct wants and goals

Contempt, the antithesis of respect, may cause your connection to disintegrate. In summary, not giving your spouse respect may undermine their self-esteem and leave them feeling irritated, unhappy, or even indifferent.

CHAPTER 2

CONNECTION

How to Establish Emotional Connection During Sex

techniques for connecting emotionally during sex:

What does being sexually attached mean? It's a physical and emotional link with your partner. Learn to cultivate this connection by connecting on a deeper level during sex.

Many couples do not pay much attention to sex and emotional connection, although both compliment one another. Here are some of the greatest suggestions on establishing a wonderful sexual connection and how to make your sex life more romantic & meaningful.

1. Foreplay and buildup

Do you desire a more fulfilling physical and emotional connection with your partner? Who doesn't?

One way you may connect emotionally during sex is by creating the atmosphere for closeness. Some fantastic suggestions for establishing the scene include giving one another massages, putting on some of your favorite sexy music, lighting candles, and clearing your calendars for sex and intimacy.

Wondering how to be more sexually intimate with your spouse or partner?

One technique to learn how to connect during sex is to establish a buildup. Tease your spouse throughout the day with dirty words, heated text messages or emails, whispers of sweet nothings and affection, and gentle touches to make them emotionally engaged before the physical deed occurs.

Building up to the occasion will make it seem more special when it eventually comes. Emotions during sex run high and keeping a connection may elevate the experience to another level entirely.

So the solution to the classic query - "how to develop emotional connection during sex" lies in large quantities of foreplay!

2. Maintain eye contact

It may seem strange at first, particularly if you're not accustomed to staring lovingly at your partner but keeping eye contact with your spouse during intimate times. It helps you connect sexually with your spouse but also helps to build your relationship.

Making eye contact during sex might make you feel vulnerable with your partner, creating sentiments of love and trust. This may lead to intense sex.

3. Talk during intercourse

One of the symptoms of an emotional connection is chatting during sex. This doesn't imply you should start debating what's for supper later.

There are two fantastic routes for communicating during sex that you might explore with your spouse. First, you may try chatting dirty to one another. You may be as graphic or as restrained as you desire with this one.

Talking during sex is a terrific way to let your inhibitions go and connect with your thoughts and dreams about being intimate with someone.

You may also adopt a more softer approach and murmur sweet nothings to one another. Tell your spouse what you appreciate about what you are doing, tell them you love them, and mention how close you feel to them.

Whatever phrases you pick, remember that chatting during sex is a method to keep your attention focused on one another during these sexually intimate times.

4. Engage in physical touch

How to get closer to your spouse sexually? When getting personal together, don't be scared to touch the areas of one another that aren't erogenous zones.

Try caressing your husband's arms or running your hands through your wife's hair throughout the deed. This will help you connect emotionally and remind you to concentrate on one another during intercourse.

5. Take care of each other's emotional needs

One key component of a good relationship is ensuring you take care of your spouse's emotional and physical needs, including intimacy and sex. Build trust and offer your spouse respect to help build emotional connection.

Give praises and tell your sweetheart of your affection.

Be fun with each other and have a regular date night. The more connected you are outside the bedroom, your sex life will be better. And the less naïve you will be about what intimate sex is. It's that easy!

6. Cuddle and kiss

Being personal before and after sex is a terrific method to establish closeness. You may achieve this by kissing regularly, a method to learn how to be more sexually intimate with your boyfriend or lover.

Kissing may be an essential component of sex and emotions in a relationship. It may help you build a profound emotional connection during sex.

Kissing is a terrific method to generate tension and connect with your partner. Kissing also raises serotonin, which helps you sleep better, enhances arousal, improves immunity, increases oxytocin and dopamine, and lessens stress.

Other techniques to promote closeness are to cuddle after sex for at least a couple of minutes, spoon before going to sleep, and perform a 6-second kiss every day before heading to work.

7. Express your love

A simple "I love" whispered at the correct moment might operate like a wonderful charm for generating an emotional connection during sex.

Expressing your affection for one other might help couples feel more connected. It might make them feel valued and appreciated. It boosts their security inside the relationship, enabling them to be more open with their spouse, especially in the bedroom.

The confidence of love may bring down the protective barriers and offer couples the opportunity to have sex with greater recklessness.

8. Giving and receiving

Maintaining a balance between how much one person within a relationship gets and provides to the other is crucial in all parts of the relationship, including sex.

To build an emotional connection during sex, ensure that you are compassionate towards your partner and emphasize their enjoyment.

9. Focus on having fun

Forming an emotional connection during sex may seem all about deep and serious feelings, but humor may assist too.

When you exchange laughter, it may help you develop relationships between you and your spouse. It may help you relax in each other's presence.

Sex does not have to be serious all the time. When you make it interesting and exciting, the link between you and your partner may grow even more intense.

10. Let your guard down

When you and your partner are having sex, the greatest thing you can do to develop an emotional connection during sex is to let your protective shield down.

Be open and eager to discover new things. Share how you feel without the fear of criticism. And don't allow yourself-protective instincts, anxieties or prior painful experiences stop you from developing a deep emotional connection during sex.

How Does Sex Affect Your Emotions? Things to Know About Attraction and Arousal

First things first: Sex implies various things to different individuals
Sex may be the ultimate expression of romantic love and connection. Or an emotional roller coaster. Or a stress reliever. Or it's all about procreation. Or it's just a good time. It can be all of these things and more.

Sex implies various things to different individuals. And whatever it means to you isn't necessarily consistent, either.

It might imply various things at different stages throughout your life, or even from one day to the next.

And you know what? It's all absolutely natural.

Despite the preconceptions, your gender has nothing to do with your emotional reaction to sex

Women are at the mercy of their roller-coaster emotions; males are firmly in control of the limited feelings they have. At least that's what common wisdom would've formerly had us think.

These notions have profound origins, yet people are far more complicated than that.

There have been some Trusted Source studies to imply that women are more outspoken about emotions, at least in the

United States and other Western European nations.

They also imply males have the same or larger physiological reaction to emotional pressures.

Some individuals need emotional attraction to feel physical attraction
Do you need to experience some amount of emotional attraction before any concept of sex enters your mind? If it sounds like you, you're certainly not alone.

Maybe you need to connect on a spiritual level. Maybe it's their thinking or the fact that you share some fundamental ideas of life.

Perhaps you felt that first flutter of excitement when they made you laugh 'til you wept.

Or it's a case of je ne sais quoi – that special something you simply can't put into words, but you know it when it occurs.

You're wanting closeness. Once your emotions are in the zone and you've created an emotional connection, you may begin to experience physical arousal.

Outside of that zone, you're simply not into sex. You're into making love.

Others find that acting on physical attraction may lead to emotional attraction Some individuals are literally pulled together like magnets.

There's a physiological response, a hunger, a totally bodily yearning for becoming physical with another person. It's a desire.

When the connection between individuals is just perfect, becoming physical may blossom into so much more.

A 2012 retrospective assessment discovered two regions of the brain that follow the passage from sexual desire to love. One is the insula. It's found in the cerebral cortex.

The other is the striatum. It's positioned within the forebrain. Interestingly, the striatum is also related to drug addiction.

Love and sexual desire stimulate various areas of the striatum.

Sex and eating are among the enjoyable things that stimulate the desire component. The process of conditioning — of reward and value — activates the love portion.

Others may discover that emotional and physical attraction function in two wholly distinct vacuums
People are complicated animals with many layers.

For some of us, there are distinct dividing lines between emotional attraction and physical attraction. They don't necessarily come together.

You could be emotionally attracted to someone without feeling the least sexual impulse. Or you have a mind-blowing physical attraction for someone who doesn't really do it for you emotionally.

Even in long-term partnerships, individuals may alternate between making love and having sex — or forgoing sexual activity completely — and that's OK.

Regardless of your particular viewpoint, sex and emotion influence the same circuits in the brain
A 2018 research shows crucial linkages between sexual, emotional, and reproductive brain processes having to do

with the endocrine system and, in particular, a hormone called kisspeptin.

According to a Tufts University neuroscience blog, sexual arousal doesn't happen in a vacuum, but in a context.

It includes cognitive, physiological, and neurological processes, all of which incorporate and are impacted by emotion. Makes sense.

What's more, most individuals feel comparable emotions during sexual activity and release
The surge of hormones involved in sex implies that some sentiments are very typical during or soon after sex.

Nobody experiences every feeling every time, of course.

Among the most favorable ones are:

- euphoria
- complete release
- relaxation and tranquility
- satisfaction
- Depending on the circumstances, you could feel certain less than favorable emotions, such as:

- vulnerability
- embarrassment
- guilt
- feeling physically or emotionally overwhelmed

If you experience postcoital dysphoria, you could even feel unhappy, worried, or crying after sex.

It's also worth remembering that sexual desire may switch down sections of the prefrontal cortex

We don't always realize it while it's happening to us, but it's evident in retrospect. It's hardly the stuff of science fiction or fantasy. It's extremely genuine.

Sexual desire may deactivate regions of the brain that let you think critically and behave like a sensible human being.

Yes, you genuinely take leave of your senses.

Oxytocin dependency is also a thing
Oxytocin is a hormone released in the brain, which opens the floodgates when you have sex.

That surge of oxytocin is involved in the physical element of sex. It may also stimulate feelings like love, affection, and joy.

It fully justifies its status as the love hormone. Alas, you might grow hooked on the emotion or downright passionate about love.

Oxytocin keeps you going back for more.

Researchers are currently dissecting the numerous factors in the desire, attraction, and attachment equation
The biochemistry of desire, attraction, and connection is far from straightforward. Hormones surely have a role.

Generally speaking, desire is fuelled by testosterone and estrogen, regardless of gender. And desire is fuelled by the yearning for sex.

Attraction is fueled by dopamine, norepinephrine, and serotonin.

Attraction may or may not entail desire, but the brain's reward center is a component. That's why you get all excited or feel like you're walking on air in a relationship's early stages.

Attachment is driven by oxytocin and vasopressin. That's what lays the basis for bonding and long-term partnerships.

There's some overlap of hormones, hormone levels vary, and there's a whole lot more to it than that.

If you wish to separate sex and emotion
There's any number of reasons why you would wish to compartmentalize sex and emotion.

It's a good idea to analyze your motivation so, if required, you can deal with any unresolved concerns.

In any case, there's no right or wrong here. You're not bound into one way of being for the rest of your life.

If you're searching for a casual relationship or a "friends with benefits" scenario, here are some suggestions:

First and foremost, be honest with the other person. It's only fair.
Talk about what you're willing — and reluctant — to offer physically and emotionally, along with what you want in return.
Discuss birth control and safe sex practices.
Work together in creating guidelines to prevent being excessively connected or reliant on each other.
Talk about what you'll do if one of you begins to desire something more.
Keep in mind that whatever your goal or as meticulous you may be, sentiments might spring up nonetheless. Emotions are strange that way.

If you wish to enhance the bond between sex and emotion

So, despite the hormones and biochemistry of it all, maybe you need something to assist enhance the link.

several methods to get started:

- Don't let sexual closeness become an afterthought, a thing you do when time allows. Schedule it. Make a date. Give it utmost importance.

- Incorporate loving contact throughout the day. Hold hands. Stroke an arm. Hug. Cuddle up. Give each other a massage. Touch doesn't always have to lead to sex straight away. A little anticipation goes a long way.

- Make eye contact and keep it. Do this regularly – when you agree, when you disagree, when you share that private joke, and when life becomes overwhelming.

Let your guard down. Be emotionally open and accessible for each other. Be their person.Kiss. Really kiss. And take your time about it.

Communicate your feelings. Say "I love you" if that's how you feel.
What turns you on? Candlelight, sensuous music, a lengthy dip in a hot tub? Whatever it is, take the time to set the setting and get in the mood.

Communicate your bodily wants. Take turns guiding each other through what you enjoy.
When things become physical, check in to your senses. Touch, see, hear, smell, and taste with every fiber of your existence.
Really be present in the moment with this individual who wants to be in the now with you. Let there be nothing else. And by all means, switch off the TV and mobile phone during your time together.

CHAPTER 3

THE DESIRE FOR SEX

Why Do We Desire Sex Or Want It.

What is Desire?

Typically, we prefer to conceive of want as an emotion — that is, emerging from our mental position, analogous to love or wrath or sadness or surprise or ecstasy. But this is probably not the case. Many scientists and psychologists now feel that desire is, in reality, a physical demand, more comparable to hunger or the blood's need for oxygen. For anybody who has been maddeningly in love, pushed to the point of despair by an insatiable need for another, this certainly doesn't sound so far-fetched. According to clinical psychologist Dr. Rob Dobrenski (denizen of shrinktalk.net), "in many respects we can't control what we want since it is a hard-wired emotional and physiological response."

Dr. Dobrenski is talking explicitly about sexual desire. No surprise: desire and sexuality are nearly inextricable. The term "desire" typically brings to mind dark romance books, adult-only activities, and a need for sexual intimacy. Sexual desire may in reality be the sole sort of want; psychoanalytic theory maintains that all other types of desire and creative energy are the consequence of misdirected sexual energy — frequently dubbed "the libido" — towards other undertakings. The biological impulse of want is exclusively sexual in origin; all else is an emotional condition grown out of this core desire.

Whether or not you accept it, it is evident that sexual desire is one of the — if not the — strongest of human wants. Typically, it takes up a big amount of our time, emotional energy, and life. Why? What fuels the seemingly unstoppable freight train of sexual desire?

Formation of Desire

According to sexologists Miss Jaiya and Ellen Heed, "desire is the coming together of visual, physiological, emotional, and biomechanical stimuli that initiate a hormonal cascade that may result in the successful fertilization of an egg by a sperm." A very clinical answer, but one embraced extensively across the profession and associated areas of research. David Buss's foundational work The Evolution of Desire: Strategies of Human Mating Is possibly the textbook on the topic. Buss says that, in essence, instincts drive our desire; the preferences we have in our sexual life are, more or less, merely an expression of our hunt for evolutionary advantage.

In the book, Buss validates a number of assumptions of conventional knowledge about sexual desire via an evolutionary appeal:

excellent looks are more essential to males than they are to women since excellent looks signify good health and consequently an improved potential to reproduce.
Women find social status crucial in a spouse since that implies a competence to care and safeguard their future offspring.
Women prefer older men because they are more likely to have the money to care for them and their children.

Buss says that these and a few more fundamental instincts drive desire and are the same across all cultures and countries. When it comes down to it, for Buss and many others, it's all about the drive to reproduce.

Obviously, Buss's approach dramatically reduces the complexity of human sexuality. Some could say that he simplifies things to the point of offending. Where, for example, do men who prefer males as sexual partners fit into this explanation? Or women who like women? And why can those who are physically unable to procreate nevertheless sense sexual desire? Nevertheless, the case is convincing.

Dr. Dobrenski agrees: "Desire is absolutely founded on an evolutionary need," he stated. "We have a very strong, often unconscious drive to propagate our species." Dobrenski puts out a crucial distinction: Perpetuating mankind is unconscious. The manifestation of sexual desire — our conscious sentiments and our performances of sexuality — is significantly more complicated than merely wishing to make kids.

The expression of sexual desire is most likely ingrained in infancy. As stress-management specialist Debbie Mandel points out, "children see their parents and absorb messages about parental sexuality and desire." Although at first we do not have the skill or the opportunity to express them, these earliest feelings of desire are not lost on us. When we hit puberty, we start to sense the evolutionary impulse towards reproduction. Immediately, this need starts to manifest itself as the acquired sexuality we have been soaking up since infancy. As we get older, it alters as it is formed by social signals from our classmates and by mass media depictions. It may take one of any number of shapes; whereas desire may be simple, sexuality is complex and varied. Sexuality is the manifestation of want, and the component of desire we can access, influence, and enjoy.

Mysteries of Desire

When the technology to look at brain activity during sexual stimulation became available, scientists anticipated it to demonstrate a pretty clear route from visual identification to emotional/sexual desire. And yet the brain-imaging studies done by Stephanie Ortigue and Francesco Bianchi-Demicheli in 2007 showed that sexual desire creates an incredibly intricate and non-linear network of brain activity, including lighting up regions in the brain typically devoted to "higher" functions, such as self-awareness and understanding others, prior to lighting up the more straightforward physical-response sections. Everything occurs exceedingly rapidly and frequently underneath the radar of awareness. In many situations, individuals do not even appear to realize what turns them on.

Attempting a scientific explanation of desire is a complicated business: Ortigue and

Bianci-Demicheli's analysis found further intricacy. The interplay of neurochemicals involved in desire is thick and intricate. And the mechanics of what may turn out to be the most crucial part of desire – phermones and cranial nerve zero – still remains unexplained. All of this uncertainty does help to explain why therapy techniques for loss of libido appear at best haphazard and sometimes useless. In many circumstances, placebos seem to function just as effectively as the genuine thing. [If you're curious, sure, Viagra works, but it doesn't truly alter desire; it affects arousal, a completely separate biological process (and a whole other debate).

The Scent of Attraction

Sexual desire itself is a force embedded deep in the stomach, acting without our consciousness and beyond our control. Jaiya and Heed think that humans are attracted to one another on a subconscious level, as the consequence of biomechanical signals, including posture and the pheromones they give out — their sexual "scent" — that drive us to pick the partners we choose. Perfume producers and ad-men have seized onto this hypothesis of pheromones, offering smells that reportedly would "help you attract sexual interest instantaneously from the other sex!" But what are they genuinely selling?

Pheromones are chemical signals given out by one member of a species in order to induce a natural reaction in another member of that same species. It's been widely noted that pheromones are utilized by animals, notably insects, to interact with one other on sublingual levels. In 1971, Dr. Martha McClintlock performed a now well-known research indicating that the menstrual cycles of women who live together in close quarters tend to become synchronized over time. McClintlock and others think this effect is generated by human female pheromone transmission and that this is merely one example of a sort of sexual communication that is continually happening between people on the sublingual level.

Jaiya and Heed, interpreting a few decades of study done by neurologist Dr. R. Douglas Fields, think that pheromones "talk to the sex regions of the brain and may stimulate a release of particular sex hormones," testosterone and estrogen. The effects of pheromones are evident in circumstances when, for example "couples who for every reason should be uninterested in one another suddenly can't stay out of each other's company after an 'up-close-and-personal encounter'" — employees on a business trip, for example.

In recent years, scientists have come to speculate that a little-known cranial nerve may be the key to the enigmatic workings of pheromones. First identified in humans in 1913, the "cranial nerve zero" or "terminal nerve" goes from the nasal cavity to the brain, finishing in what Dr. Fields calls "the hot-button sex areas of the brain." For years, scientists assumed that nerve zero was part of the olfactory nerve, helping our brain process odors. But in 2007, Dr. Fields revealed that although the brain of a pilot whale had no olfactory nerve whatsoever, it did have nerve zero. What difference does a whale brain make? Whales long ago evolved to lose the sense to smell, their nostrils becoming blowholes. And yet, whereas whales no longer have neural machinery for smell, they still have nerve zero, linking the whale's blowhole to its brain. Dr Fields undertook several tests, revealing that activating nerve zero produced instinctive sexual reactions in animals.

Dr. Fields, along with many others, now think that cranial nerve zero may be involved for deciphering the signals of sex pheromones and triggering reproductive activity. In other words, cranial nerve zero may be the bio-machinery for desire.

A Potent Cocktail

Pheromones may operate as a form of stoplight for sexual desire. They let us know that we're good to go, but they obviously don't work alone. Regardless of what switched it on, something's still got to be driving the automobile. It turns out to be an intoxicating cocktail of hormones and neurochemicals activating in the brain.

That "hot-button sex region" identified by Dr. Fields is the septal nucleus, which, among other things, regulates the release of the two principal sex hormones in the body: testosterone and estrogen. Both hormones are necessary in the process of desire. Scientists know this, since as men get older, they tend to lose testosterone and, as a consequence, experience erection and libido difficulties. Women also lose testosterone as they age. However, owing to unsatisfactory results from research involving testosterone administration in women with a lack of sexual drive, experts now feel that a mix of testosterone and estrogen is the ultimate "love hormone."

Estrogen and testosterone, in turn, increase neurochemicals in the brain — particularly, dopamine, serotonin, norepinephrine and oxytocin. Dr. Craig Malkin, a clinical psychologist who is now authoring a book on how humans govern desire, remarked that the effect of this neurochemical cocktail may be tremendous. "The mix of neurochemicals creates dizzying emotions of exhilaration, ecstasy, and passion," he stated. "Some brain imaging studies suggest a resemblance between neural activity in patients with obsessive-compulsive disorder and those who are falling in love." Love – or at least desire — actually drives you insane. How? What are these chemicals truly doing? **Dopamine** - Dopamine has largely been examined in the context of drug addiction.

Essentially, it's the neurotransmitter that makes external stimuli stimulating. Dopamine educates you to connect the sense of being filled and pleasured with particular items. In the case of sexual desire, dopamine is produced in the brain anytime you meet something to which or someone to whom you're attracted.

Serotonin - Serotonin is comparable to dopamine; it is a neurotransmitter that teaches your body a cycle of desire and fulfillment.

Norepinephrine - Usually, this neurotransmitter is activated when we need more energy to flee a hazardous or terrifying scenario. But it also tends to grow during masturbation and intercourse, peaking at climax and then falling.

Oxytocin: Oxytocin has been termed the "cuddle hormone." It is considered to play a vital role in parent-child bonding and in couple development. A 1992 research by the National Institute of Mental Health of the prairie vole – an animal noted for being strongly monogamous — found that while creating a relationship with a partner, the vole's brain produces a surge of oxytocin. Even more interesting, when oxytocin is inhibited, the vole can't create a link at all. Oxytocin doesn't produce arousal, but it may be part of the broader drive that is desired. According to Dr. Malkin, it "relaxes our guard and increases trust."

Various research over the years have revealed that all of these neurochemicals and more (including epinephrine, alpha melanocyte polypeptide, phenethylamine, and gonadotropins), are in one way or another involved with sexual desire. But when it comes down to it, it's very much impossible to isolate any one process.

It's good to take a short step back to observe why.

CHAPTER 4

SEX EXPLORATION

What Should we try next

Imagine you're on a date with someone who's captivated your sexual attention. The discussion got flirtatious a while ago, and both of you are riding the wave of that exhilaration. Suddenly they lean in and say, "So, what are you into?"

Your heart beats, and a rushing sound fills your ears. Your brain swims with potential replies. What am I into? What sex stuff thrills me? If you've never taken the time for sexual exploration, you may not have an answer that is true to your identity and reflects your ideals regarding sexual activity.

When you're masturbating, it's crucial to understand what your body enjoys and how your sexual arousal cycle works. When you love sex with a partner, you want to share your wants. You need sexual exploration. Read on for some advice on sexual exploration and how it might enhance your sex life.

What is sexual exploration?

Sexual exploration is the age-appropriate investigation of bodily parts and sexual desire. It generally begins in early infancy when youngsters find that caressing their private areas feels wonderful. During adolescence and beyond, sexual exploration might involve masturbation or consenting partnered sexual behavior.

Sexual exploration is a healthy component of human growth. People participate in sexual exploration to explore their body, find out what forms of touch result in sexual stimulation (and what doesn't), and even to help figure out their sexual orientation and gender identity.

However, if persons face humiliation for touching their genitals or endure sexual violence, they may not feel comfortable with sexual exploration. Most sex education programs don't explore sexual exploration beyond stating sexual desire. The lack of understanding and a culture of secrecy around sexuality may impede healthy sexual development.

Sexual discovery should continue throughout your lives. Young adults may have different sexual demands than teenagers, which will keep altering as they mature. Your sexual requirements might fluctuate depending on your life stage, the flexibility of sexual orientation, or even sickness or injury. Exploration is the way to stay up with your body.

What are the advantages of sexual exploration?

Not only may sexual exploration help you answer the question "what are you into?" on a date, it can open up new worlds for you. People that participate in sexual exploration know what they enjoy and don't. Sexual exploration is the key to building a sexual connection (with yourself or with others) that fits your needs and resonates with your ideals.

Sexual exploration enables you to share your needs with a companion or utilize them to make your alone sessions so pleasant you don't waste time hunting for a mate. Exploration helps you learn how to recognize sexual sensations, start sexual encounters, and discuss sexual preferences without shame.

What is the difference between sexual exploration and sexual experimentation?

Sexual exploration entails approaching masturbation and sharing sexual encounters with an attitude of curiosity. You're investigating bodies and feelings and attempting to construct a vision of what a fulfilling sex life looks like for you. Sexual exploration makes your sexual health a crucial aspect of your well-being and helps you identify and negotiate sexual sensations and participate in proper decision-making during sexual relationships.

Experimenting is trying something out to see what occurs. People commonly use sexual experimentation to characterize acts considered promiscuous or prohibited. As long as the sexual experimentation or exploration you're engaged in is consensual, safe, and with age-appropriate partners, there is no such thing as promiscuity or forbidden sexual activities. Sexual experimentation is sexual exploration. Explore or explore as you desire and with whoever you want to, whether that's queer partners, threesomes, non-monogamy, mild bondage, breath play, pegging, or something else.

How do individuals explore their sexuality? Sexual fantasies, viewing or listening to erotic stimuli, talking and exploring sexual desire, and even shared sexual encounters may be curiosity-driven activities aimed to help you learn more about your body and your partner's body.

Masturbation

Sexual exploration frequently begins with masturbation and other self-touch. But don't panic if you've had sexual intercourse and never masturbated. It's never too late to start!

Rather than rushing to climax, start gently and enchant yourself. Use candles, music, or other components to produce an environment that awakens all your senses. Dance or explore your nude body in front of a mirror. Let the look and feel of your body turn you on. Experiment with a variety of erogenous zones, various postures, styles of touch, and sex toys to find out what you prefer.

Shared sexual experiences

You may explore your sexuality via consenting sexual interactions with someone you trust. Positive sexual experiences may help you find out if you love giving and receiving oral sex, have any interest in anal sex, prefer intercourse to other sorts of sex, or desire sexual activity that doesn't require penetration.

If you're participating in sexual exploration with a partner it's preferable to conceive of your experience as sexual play. This may be tough to commence, particularly in a society that focuses so strongly on heteronormative penis-in-vagina intercourse. But sex is intended to be enjoyable and lively, and partnered sexual exploration is an excellent way to retain that emphasis.

Try initiating a discussion regarding sexual play with your spouse by discussing something you're interested about. For example, "I heard about nipple play leading to orgasms for some individuals and want to try it. Tonight, can we get some massage oil and attempt various forms of nipple play?" Phrasing what you desire as an offer to explore, rather than a refusal of intercourse, may enable your partner to more quickly accept your request for sexual exploration.

Sexual fantasy

Before you can construct (or rebuild) the sex life you desire, you may visualize it.

Fantasizing is an amazing start to sexual exploration. Sexual fantasy may be especially potent for persons questioning their sexual or gender identity.

Try enjoying erotica depicting same-sex and opposite-sex pairings. Which one gets you going more? Maybe you'll find a sexual attraction in both genders! Enjoying a certain sort of erotica doesn't imply you're gay or straight, but it may be a place to start exploring, especially if you've only been in romantic relationships with individuals of one gender.

Sexual fantasy may also deepen your exploration with a partner. Try reading erotica together or exchanging sexual fantasies with questions geared to get you chatting about what you'd want to try. You may discover you have certain sexual desires you've never addressed that take your sex life to the next level.

Inspiration for your sexual adventure

Sexual exploration begins with curiosity about your body and the range of sexual experiences accessible. Sexual exploration should be a frequent element of your sexual wellness practice. Your sexual interests, tastes, and requirements will vary over time, and if you stop experimenting, you may lose out on some wonderful possibilities for pleasure.

The bottom line: Sexual exploration may be a wonderful method to strengthen your connection with your spouse. It may be that merely expressing your sexual hobbies enhances trust and communication, or that the novelty of attempting new activities and getting to know each other on various levels fosters deeper closeness. Remember that your sexual wants, hobbies, fetishes, and fantasies aren't anything to be embarrassed of and exploring these things may really enrich your relationship.

The Beauty Of Sex

CHAPTER 5

PRIORITIZE SEX

When Dara and Kevin were in premarital counseling, their pastor asked them to describe five habits or personality characteristics about the other person that they found unpleasant. Dara gazed at her blank piece of paper and added, "Honestly, nothing about Kevin irritates me."

By their 10-year anniversary her gripe list had expanded, mostly due to the burden of managing two kids, a hard career, a gigantic mortgage, and an incontinent cat. These made even the slightest disagreements between her and Kevin enormous annoyances, and left her little energy for sex.

Every couple hopes the passion and starry-eyed love could endure forever. But at some time every husband and wife must cross the invisible line between dream love and actual reality, where the majority of marriage is lived out.

Even King Solomon and the Shulammite crossed that line when difficulties threatened to damage their intimacy: "Catch for us the foxes, the small foxes that wreck the vines, our vineyards that are in blossom" (Song of Songs 2:15). She informed him, "We've had troubles. Can't you see those tiny foxes? They're going to wreck everything for us. Do something about this."

Most Old Testament scholars feel that the vines in this line symbolize Solomon and the Shulammite's love. Everything appears ideal, except that she notices several small foxes in their vineyard, and notifies Solomon of their existence. While appearing innocent, foxes excavated tunnels and channels that disturbed the soil surrounding the vines, preventing them from building a permanent root system. In this situation, that root system is their closeness.

Proverbial emblems of destruction, the tiny foxes in this verse reflect the minor issues that eat at the base of their love.

We must capture those foxes that eat at the base of our love, because if we don't, they'll kill our desire for sexual connection.

A recent cover of Newsweek portrayed a husband and wife in bed, clad in full-length pajamas. He looks blankly at a computer on his lap as she shovels spoonfuls of Häagen-Dazs into her lips, a zoned-out expression on her face. A blazing headline says, "No Sex, Please, We're Married." The subtitle questions, "Are Stress, Kids, and Work Killing Romance?"

The answer? Yes! Stress is eating us alive. And the two most prevalent foxes, or intimacy killers, for married couples? Work and kids.

Intimacy Stealer #1: Overwork

Work, work, work. According to former Labor Secretary Robert Reich, Americans worked 350 hours more this year than previous year, and this increasing trend continues. And the outcome is neglected marriages.

John works 75 hours a week under the pretense of providing for his family. Amy's call for him to spend more time at home awakens great emotion in them both. He's angry: "Doesn't she realize the strain I'm under?" She's despondent: "Doesn't he understand he's becoming a stranger to me?"

Men are not the only ones who suffer from overwork. Women who are working full time are frequently still the primary family and home managers. And don't forget about stay-at-home parents.

Lynne is a stay-at-home parent. You'd think she'd have time on her hands, yet she homeschools their five children, runs the household, teaches Sunday school, and sells cosmetics on the side.

If you asked Lynne, "How's your sex life?" she'd replied, "Sex—what's that?"

It used to be that many times a year, Americans took a vacation. They fled to a lovely cottage (with no television) beside a mountain lake, where they drank lemonade, listened to the katydids chirp, and appreciated the opportunity to get away from the phone and their daily routine. These days, instead of going away, we carry it all with us. On our previous trip, we each brought a mobile phone and a laptop. Count it up: between us, five days away with four mobile phones, four computers, two Palm Pilots, and two Day-Timers.

Unfortunately, continual contact with the outside world might leave us isolated from our companions.

Intimacy Stealer #2: Children

First you married, then you had kids. Problems occur when couples reverse this sequence. We best serve our kids when we make our marriage our primary focus. Children, although blessings from God and a delight to parents, demand ongoing care, decreasing possibilities for closeness. Cassie informed us: "I've got three preschoolers. I'm so fatigued with kids dragging on me all day that by evening, I can scarcely move. Then my spouse wants sex, and he wonders why I'm upset. The last thing I need is another person dragging on my worn-out body."

Murphy's Law states, "Sex creates small babies. Kids have little sex."

Jody and Linda: Years ago, when our kids were toddlers, we decided we needed some time alone as a couple. After years of being pregnant and breastfeeding, Linda was beyond fatigued. So we booked a weekend away. We found a lady to stay with our children. Everything was in place—and then the babysitter became ill. So we planned a second holiday. Again, we spent days putting every detail in place—then Linda became ill. On our third effort, we thought, Surely this time it will happen—and the vehicle broke down. Our efforts to be alone were adding additional stress to our already stressed-out life, but we were determined to spend time together, without kids. On the fourth attempt we had our weekend away. It was magnificent, well worth battling for.

Steal It Back!

In our busy, stress-filled lives, we race from job to children to marriage, and in our hurry, we wind up putting out fires rather than living by priority. One couple expressed it this way: "We keep saying we'll find time for us—next year will be different, the kids will be older, job responsibilities will be different. We've been stating these things for five years and nothing has changed. We've finally understood we must find time now, this week, not next year."

Perhaps part of the issue is our viewpoint. It isn't about finding time; it's about creating time.

So what do we do about employment and kids? How can we catch these foxes and recover intimacy?

1. Talk to God. If your heart isn't right, you'll disregard how to spend more time with each other with an indifferent shrug, and a "No, I don't want to do that." The beginning point to generating time for your partner is to ask God to establish in you a desire to make your sex life a top priority.

2. Schedule time on your calendars. Sit down together with your calendars. Across the top of a sheet of paper, write the name of each family member, establishing a column for each. List the activities linked with each individual, and how much time that activity takes each week. Be careful to include transportation time as well as time spent in planning or preparing for the activity. Your objective is to assess all your present activities so you can recover at least two hours a week and one weekend a yeaso r that the two of you can spenime alone together. To attain this aim, you'll need to remove or reduce some activities on your list. Review each activity and ask these questions: Can this be omitted from our schedule? If so, how can we reduce its drain on our time? Discuss how you can take two hours a week to concentrate on each other, and write down that time on your agenda.

3. Interview an elderly couple. Invite for supper one or two older couples whose marriages you appreciate. Ask them questions such as: How did you maintain your marriage aas priority? How did you create time for intimacy? What's your most memorable romantic moment together? What advice do you have for us as a couple? Is there anything you'd alter about the importance you put on your relationship?

Their insights will motivate you to build marriage minutes together.

4. Brainstorm with couples your age. Organize a "Potluck With a Purpose" and invite couples that also desire time together. Ask every couple to be prepared to discuss three unique ways they've done to seize marital minutes. Compile a master list and ask the couples if they're prepared to meet every six months (or year) to update the list.

5. Fast from television for one week. You'll be astonished hat ow much time you'll have for romance when you switch off the tube. Try it for one week and notice the difference it makes in finding time to enjoy your closeness.

6. Hire a babysitter. Don't squander your babysitting bucks on going to watch a movie! Instead, hire a sitter to take your kids to a park Saturday morning for two hours while you spend that time at home—in bed.

7. Schedule a motel date. When inquisitive teens pack the home and won't go to bed until midnight, it might short circuit their love life. Leave your teenagers with a pizza and a decent movie, pack a picnic basket stocked with fun food, a CD player, candles, and scented lotion, and head to a hotel from 5-11 p.m. You'll be shocked by how much loving and chatting you can accomplish with no ringing phones! It's cheaper than supper out and a movie— and more fun!

8. Enjoy the Sabbath relaxation. God wants us to take a Sabbath break. Our bodies were intended for a day of relaxation once a week. We urge you to work and perform things with your kids for six days but then take off one day. No work. No shopping. No running to sporting activity. Instead, set aside the whole day to worship God, take naps, relax, and play together. This is part of intimacy—finding rest in each other, resting in each other's arms, and enjoying the proximity without the stress of life.